Unravel the Veil

Maria Kitsios, LMT

Edited by Jaclyn Reuter
Cover Design by Danijela Mijailovic
Formatting by Tapioca Press

ISBN: 978-1-7378369-2-6 (paperback)
ISBN: 978-1-7378369-3-3 (eBook)

Publisher email address: mkitsios8@gmail.com

Printed by Maria Kitsios, in the United States of America.

First printing edition 2021

Dedicated to all those along the path
of my journey to Source
who helped me see clearer
and showed me the way
towards unraveling the veil
of my own Intuition.

INTRODUCTION

The Third Eye Chakra
According to the Vedas (ancient Indian sacred texts), the physical body is composed of seven main energy or vortex centers called chakras. Chakra is the Sanskrit word for wheel.
The seven main chakras run along the spine-beginning from the root and ending with the crown chakra.

1. Root
2. Sacral
3. Solar plexus
4. Heart
5. Throat
6. Third eye
7. Crown

Each chakra has a different color, element, sound, mantra, function, location, major organ, and association. The flow or blockage/imbalance of subtle energy in each chakra determines the health or disease of the individual body.

This book is the second of a series of seven poetry books.

It is composed of poems associated with topics of the third eye chakra. The third eye is the sixth chakra. It is the one associated with our Intuition, vision, inner wisdom and knowing.

Third Eye Chakra information:
Sanskrit name: Ajna
Color: Indigo
Element: Light
Sound: Om
Mantra: "I See"
Practice: Visualization meditation
Function: Knowing, intuition and insight, inner vision
Location: Between the eyebrows slightly above eye level
Organ: Pineal gland, eyes, nose, ears, brain, nervous system
Associations: Emotional intelligence, Truth, openness to new ideas, psychic abilities
Dysfunctions when imbalanced: Nightmares, blurred vision, deafness, headaches, seizures, learning disabilities, and doubting your inner wisdom.

1. WATCHED

Life is a movie being watched by the observer who
laughs and laughs and laughs.
Laughter and amusement
for the silly nature of humanity.
A silliness shown in our stubborn insistence
on being serious all the time!

2. MOVIE UNFOLDING

Be present.
Life is a movie unfolding,
yet we are too distracted
to sit and watch it.
We are the audience
who needs to simply
enjoy the movie
without thinking it reality.

3 . GLANCE

I looked upon the vast sky and saw my Self.
I glanced upon the grey clouds, the thunderstorm,
and drops of rain and saw my sorrow.
I looked upon the endless sky and saw my Self.
I glanced upon the sun's rays reflecting on the water
and saw my smile.
I looked upon the rivers and the mountains,
the woods and the desert.
I glanced upon the stars at night and the shadows in the day.
I looked everywhere to find beauty and I saw it in my Self.

4. MAKE LIGHTER

Enlighten: to make lighter
by releasing all which holds us
down and back.
To let go of heaviness
in order to embody the light.
A physical, mental, and spiritual letting go.
To live an unattached life,
ready to leave in any given moment
because nothing holds us
here, there, anywhere.
We are free.

5. LIGHTEN

Open your heart with a hug and lighten your face with a smile.

6. BE LIGHT

Even a small amount of light
causes darkness to disappear.
This is the power of light!
Be light and enlighten.

Our presence is a plug which recharges our spiritual battery.
It elevates and heals us both-
unblocking stuck energy channels in our bodies.
It flows with such ease-
opening up horizons of growth for each of us.
Our meetings are aligned by the Universe
and so, we see again.
Going and coming as another guide to the next level
of Enlightenment and to Source.

8. GUIDES

When you have vision and trust your Intuition-
you naturally flow with it.
Life is always teaching us,
always guiding us when we open up to the Universe's wisdom.
Stay blessed to witness
and be open enough to understand
the signs.

Feelings are as dangerous as thoughts
because of their uncontrollable,
changing nature.
It is unwise to interpret reality through them.
We must use our Intuition to make decisions and find answers.
Intuition is the best guide.
But first, we must train ourselves to hear its voice
through feelings' loud noise.

10. MEDIUMS

I now know my life path
because the Universe led me to it
through some amazing mediums.

How small we are,
we, who think ourselves enormous!
Tell me,
how small are we
who view the "I" important.
If we could only see
that this "I" is blinding us,
then maybe we could trust
the Eye that's guiding us.

How small are we
who think the ego is all there is!
Tell me,
how small are we
who choose to live like this.
We truly are significant-
not due to our human form,
but for being Specks of the Divine
yearning to go back home.

12. THE EYE

Everything in this world
revolves around the "I".
So, by now
you'd think none of us
would be blind.
And if it weren't for this
we'd surely break down
as a majority and die.
But sometimes this "I"
tells us to look outside the self
into something greater.
So, go ahead and
offer your Eye to the world.
The blindness in humanity
is hideous.

13. EYES

A person's eyes never age.
The spark within the heart
shines brighter through them
every day.
Regardless of how many
his years may be.
A heart that loves, laughs,
gives, and dreams is eternal
in the Spirit of a child.
If you desire endless youth,
stay humble
and stay kind
each moment of your life.

14. THIRD EYE

Don't tell me
you want to be stupefied
just because reality
is a lie.

Don't tell me you lost your Will
to live or die.
Close your eyes and come
open your Third Eye.

Don't you know-
there's latent wisdom within?
It patiently awaits,
right beneath your skin.

So, don't whisper
such foolish words to me.
I've been blinded before,
but now I see.

So come, my friend,
join in celebration!
Let's rejoice in the love
and light of Creation!

15. THIRD EYE/PINEAL GLAND AWAKENING

Let us tap into our psychic abilities
and our True Self.
Our truest power of manifestation and Abundance lays latent
awaiting our Awakening.
Empaths, light workers,
men and women of medicine-
Let us unite in prayer and in Love.
Let us offer guidance through the dark times
like a lantern in a tunnel.
Let us give our hands to those befallen to grief and sorrow,
giving them courage to stand again.
Let us always give of ourselves
in the humblest way,
knowing our godliness.
Let us be a mirror of the Divine
and show each other our grandest Self.
Let us remain strong warriors
battling lower frequencies
of negative thought
and elevate ourselves with every breath.
Breath is life.
So let us take a moment to collectively breathe together tonight.
Let the Intention of our breath
be to fill our body

with Divine light on every inhalation-
filling the invisible space of aura
with Abundance and Love,
expanding with each exhale-
filling up the world.

16. JESUS

In the scriptures,
when Jesus was healing the blind
and restoring their vision
(third eye chakra)
after he disappeared for several years
(where he went into solitude and learned to meditate)
he was performing Reiki.
Just as the Buddha sat under a tree in isolation
to obtain Enlightenment.
Each of us is capable of all this!
If only we grow to embrace
solitude and meditation.
We need to understand the power within us.
These men were like you and I.
We're all part of the Divine.
The difference is that they knew
the nature of the Universe
and understood energy.

17. YOUR MIND

I want to read your mind
and share with the world
all the beauty therein I find.

18. VIEW THE PEOPLE

View all the people around you
as if they are to die soon
because they might.
If you see this reality-
you cannot hate anyone.

19. L.I.F.E.

When you look around
with vision of the "I",
you start to see into
the illusion of reality.
Look to understand
the temporary state
of this Mayan place
born from Samsara-
one of a seemingly
limiting and challenging nature-
until you look around
with clearer vision and see
with deeper eyes.
To know of our eternal existence
is a freeing, yet painful act of acceptance-
an awareness to go
and let go.
See the Truth of who this "I" is
and know life is an acronym for
Let It Flow Easily.

20. INTENT

Let us be more conscious and aware
of the choices we make.
Let us understand the reasons we make them.
Let us be more open to acting out of love
rather than any other Intention.

21. THEY ALL HOLD ENERGY

Words, thoughts-
they all hold energy.
Raise your vibration,
expand your frequency.
Live the life you were brought here to live-
a life filled with Abundance.

Trust the wisdom of the Universe and take a road less travelled.
The road to success is usually rocky, solitary,
and without many trails
because few have the courage to embark upon it.
Be the minority and take that journey.
Your soul will appreciate it greatly.
Trust in your inner voice and forge ahead courageously.

23. INTUITION

Words, thoughts, and emotions
blind us more often than not.
We see better while being present and in flow.
All is revealed
through Intuition.

24. INTENTION

There is greater depth to each person
than what is seen with faded vision.
You need to dive into the realm of his existence
to know anything about him.
To see the distant stars in the sky-
you must wholeheartedly focus on them.
To see any beauty in this world-
you must always do the same.

Open up to the magic of energy.
Open up to your own magic
which lays latent inside.
Untapped potential.
Create in the metaphysical realm and attract Abundance.
It exists all around us.
Heal and love.
Open up your heart!

26. OUR SENSITIVITY

Our introversion and our sensitivity are our beauty.
They are our Intuition,
our spirituality and our knowing.
The childlike spirit which lives on always,
alive within us.

27. KNOW SELF

A different version of us
exists in our various interactions.
We choose which side of ourselves
we prefer
by the company we keep.
Which is your favorite side of you?
To know anything,
we first must know ourselves.

28. NATURALLY FLOW

When you have vision and trust your Intuition,
you naturally flow with it.

29. TRUTH IS LIGHT

Truth is never harsh,
though your judgement might make it seem so.
Upon hearing it for the first moment
it might feel heavy-
simply because it tears down your ego.
But if you take time to think about it,
Truth is always light!

30. TRUTH CANNOT BE LABELED

Truth cannot be labeled
or measured
or confined
in foolish terms such as
any religious dogma or deity.
Truth is simply
all around us
in the metaphysical world
and some of us are open to
seeing and feeling it.
You too will come to such
realizations on your own.
I believe everyone does
in his or her own time.
The spirit always finds its way
when the eyes are ready
to see its beauty.

We smile, we cry,
we yell, we kneel.
We dance, we sing,
we heal.
The process of unveiling
the surreal.
Dissolving illusion
forces us to feel.

32. SEE YOU

Not everyone you encounter will see you,
understand you, or appreciate you.
And that is okay.
You don't need to prove yourself to others.
As long as you know who you are and your values are strong,
your life will be prosperous and blessed.
Shine on, my bright beings!

33. SEE CLEARLY

I see clearly.
I listen to my Intuition.
I trust my Intuition
and am guided by my vision.
Amen.

34. PURE

I want to touch the world
with warm hands
and see it with pure eyes.

35. NEW YEAR

Life is a precious, fleeting
blessing.
Each moment is a new year.
Each day is a new life.
We must grow and adapt
with each rising and setting
of the sun.

36. STAY BLESSED

Life is always teaching us,
always guiding us when we open up to the Universe's wisdom.
Stay blessed
and open to witness
the messages.

37. WISEST QUALITY

Humbleness is the Divine's wisest quality.

38. WITH WISDOM

With wisdom comes the Truth,
the Will to understand it,
and the Courage to continue living in this world.

39. ADVENTURE

A day that is lacking in adventure and laughter
is a dull day.
So, dance for no reason
because your heart wants to dance.
Laugh at your silliness and childishness
because only the ignorant are serious all the time.
Dip deeper and deeper into the meaning behind all things
because that's an adventure of the mind.
Hug and kiss others
because you are here to give of yourself.
Make conversation with a random stranger at the laundromat
because everyone has something to teach you.
When you pay attention to each moment,
each one becomes an adventure.
So, focus and you will see clearly.

40. OUT AT THE STREAMS

Looking out into those streams
you view your wildest dreams.
They seem so near, yet traveling-
as the ocean's waves keep battling.
So are you and so am I
to reach this life before we die.
That day will come before the end
when you'll be in the dream, my friend.

41. UNIVERSAL ENERGY

We're a small Speck
in the enormous Universe(s).
This is the only certainty.
Yet, we find ourselves
overwhelmed and pressured often-
as if we were of great importance,
but we are so tiny
and insignificant.
Even so,
that little insignificant energy ball
is a part of a larger picture.
That is what makes us valuable
in some mysterious way.
We are a piece of the Universal energy-
the Wholeness of God.

42. WE ARE ALL CONNECTED

We are all connected
on a deep and very real level.
You and I and the entire Universe.
This entire realm of Existence is one.
To believe anything else is to look only at
the superficial levels of being.
For a spiritual and philosophical mind
that is not possible.

43. EXTRA YEARS

People are scared of death,
but most don't make good use of the time they are alive.
You don't want to die tomorrow,
but what will you do with twenty extra years?
Will you be of service to others?
Will you create and manifest for the Greatest Good?
Will the years granted to you
make any difference at all?

It's important to take time
and reflect on the past.
Reflect on the inner workings
of your being.
Reflect on who you are
and what you want in your life.
Reflect on the things you attract
and those you resist.
Reflect, understand, and only then
can you grow from all the hardships.
Only then will you learn necessary lessons,
break the chains of your conditionings.
gain self-knowledge and wisdom,
and move forward into a future that mirrors
your heart's desire.
Reflect, reflect, reflect!
Stop resisting happiness.

45. REFLECTION

Mirrors-
that's what we are-
shattered and broken
on the floor.
We see pieces of ourselves
in scattered reflection.
Naked, vulnerable,
lacking protection.
Mirrors-
is all we are-
torn down,
wall and door.
Allowing ourselves
to be seen
and bringing wreckage
to the scene.
Seeing pieces of reflection
on the ground.
In awe at beauty
we have found.
Mirrors-
that's what we are-
shattered and broken
on the floor.

46. MIRROR

I am a mirror.
We are all mirrors-
mirrors of soul.
We reflect and project
onto one another
who we are.
Mirrors of frustration,
unresolved inner battles
with fear, hate, and anger.
Throwing cold rocks,
thus shattering one another.
And with bare hands
struggling to gather
broken pieces of glass
from the floor.
Cutting through flesh,
time and again.
Yet,
seeing the blood ooze out
we feel no disgust at our
pathetic condition.
No pain.
For we have become so numb-
we cannot even bear
to look at ourselves

without being torn to shreds.
Shattering mirrors-
this is all we do
to each other.
All of us,
so-called civilized,
intelligent beings.

47. MIRROR IN THE WORLD

The greatest mirror in the world
is our life's creation.

48. NEVER-ENDING
NIGHTMARE

This life without a dream
would be a never-ending nightmare.

49. GLANCING AT A SCREEN

We, humans, no longer look at each other.
We don't see each other's faces.
We miss out on so much because we try to fill voids
by using social media as a means for temporary validation,
an escape from boredom of routine in a life we are unhappy with.
Instead of working on improving this precious life-
we waste it glancing into a screen all day and night.
It's truly a disease.
Weakened new age world!

50. LYRICS OF THE BLIND

We'd be able to see better
if we were blind.
Use abstract vision
of the Third Eye
to look inside
unknown colors
and traced shapes-
sensing touch
and predicting fate.
We'd be able to see better
if we were blind
for every day we witness
hate crimes of all kind.
We forget to see
that we, humans, are all alike
despite looks,
race, age, weight, or height.
We'd be able to see better
if we were blind.

51. SOUVENIRS OF WAR

Save the photographs-
soon they might be gone.
The scissors of time
seem to find a way
to cut through the memories.
Ripping your past
to tiny pieces of a nothing.
Do me the favor
and save the photographs.
Hide them away
in the deepest place,
the darkest corner of your mind.
Hide them away
somewhere the shadows can't crawl.
Hold them as souvenirs of war.

52. AN ABYSS

The human psyche is an abyss.
So much depth, darkness, confusion
lays dormant within each of us.
Who can ever see us so clearly
in this dark place?
The human psyche is an abyss.
An abyss to get lost in,
to delve into and explore,
to become consumed by
and to lovingly embrace.

53. I STAY AWAKE ALL NIGHT AND THINK ABOUT MY LIFE

My eyes are getting weary
and my body's aching with fatigue,
but my mind keeps racing
and now I feel so weak.
I can't bring myself to lay
and fall right on asleep.

I stay awake all night
and think about my life.

Friends are, but a few
so to silence I thus spoke
and I'll be falling down to sleep
when all the world has woke.

I stay awake all night
and think about my life.

Again I view tomorrow
turn into today
and thus, my restless body
in stillness cannot stay.

I stay awake all night
and think about my life.

Night, take me with you
and hide me within your darkness.
Hide me from the fake glances of man.
I don't want to view broken smiles
and useless grins.
Night, take me away
for I no longer want to live here
and as a Mother-
you alone-
understand me every time.
Hold me in your arms
and never let me go.
Save my soul
from the weak.
Shine your light of mystery upon me
for this is what binds us together
in Eternity.

55. END OF THE TUNNEL

There is a light at the end of the tunnel
and that light is within you.
You can only see it
with the soul's Eye.

~ACKNOWLEDGMENTS~

I want to express my gratitude for everyone who made this book possible.

Thank you to my editor, Jaclyn Reuter.

Thank you to my formatter, Nola Li Barr.

Thank you to my cover designer, Danijela Mijailovic.

Thank you to family. Such a sacred word and bond. Thank you to my mother, Galatia Kitsios. Your intuitive nature has always inspired me to trust my own and to listen to its subtle voice as it speaks to me often. Thank you to my brother, Spiro Kitsios. Your quiet reserve and wisdom have helped me many times with much needed advice. Thank you to my father, Ioannis Kitsios. You are my angel and I will continue to connect with you as I look beyond the veil which seemingly separates us. I am grateful to feel your presence with me still.

Thank you to all of my friends, close and far. You make life more enjoyable and your continued support and love are irreplaceable for me. I am grateful to have encountered amazing beings on this sacred life journey to Source.

Thank you to my beautiful friend, Magda Katirtzoglou. Our connection is third eye based and we understand one another on a higher level than most. I enjoy the moments we reach out to one another simultaneously. Continue to trust your inner knowing and remain grateful for the visions which arrive through your dreams. Your compassionate and nurturing nature is a blessing. You are a gift to this world and to me.

Thank you to my brother from another, Constantine Economides. You remind me to stay focused on the important things and guide me back to myself if ever I stray into the darker side. Thank you for your patience and support. Our friendship means a lot to me.

Thank you to Leslie Ann Garnes. The Universe brings certain people into our lives at precise moments. Your presence is such a Divine encounter. I am grateful we found our way to each other. You encourage me to embrace myself and see the light within me. Thank you for being such an awesome friend. I am grateful for you.

Thank you to Vicky Bi. From the first moment we met, I knew we were sisters. Wise beyond your years, you are an old soul. I find myself constantly learning from you. You remind me of my younger self in so many ways and I will always be here for you.

Thank you to my sweet love, Raf. The tenderness and compassion in our interactions fill my heart with joy and my mind with peace. I will honor our sacred bond always.

My gratitude goes out to everyone who has been a part of my healing journey and this incredible opportunity (life) for spiritual evolution.

May we always see the light within each other. Namaste.

Join Maria's newsletter and receive a free copy of the asanas guideline.

www.subscribepage.com/thejourneytosourceasanas

Maria Kitsios is a New York licensed massage therapist and a Reiki master since 2013. Before dedicating her life to these healing modalities, she obtained a bachelor's degree in Behavioral Science. In 2021, she became a certified yoga instructor. Through many years of meditation, physical fitness, massage, and energy work, she has discovered several truths about the mind/body/spirit connection on the deepest levels. Her first published book is *The Journey to Source*. *The Journey to Source* is composed of poems associated with the crown chakra and is the first of the series of seven books. It was published on September 14, 2021. *Unravel the Veil* is the second book of the same series.

Instagram: @mkitsioslmt
Facebook: @Maria Kitsios, LMT